THIS JOURNAL BELONGS TO:

_____

_____

COPYRIGHT © 2019 BY AGILE EXPRESSIONS

ALL RIGHTS RESERVED. NO PART OF THIS BOOK MAY BE REPRODUCED OR USED IN ANY MANNER WITHOUT WRITTEN PERMISSION OF THE COPYRIGHT OWNER.

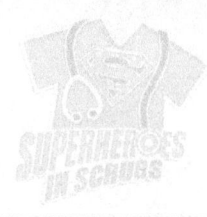

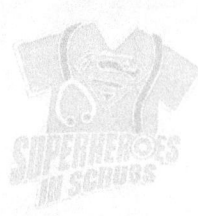

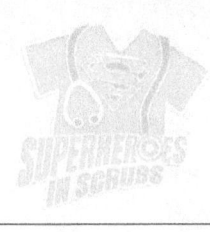

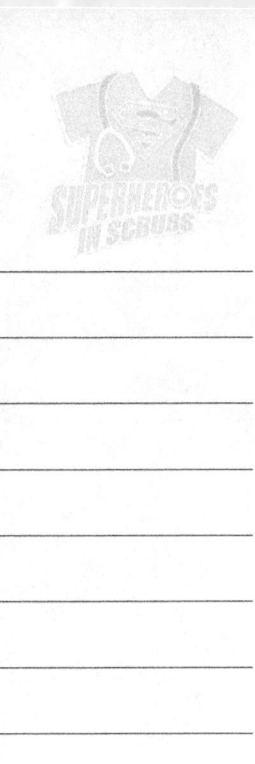

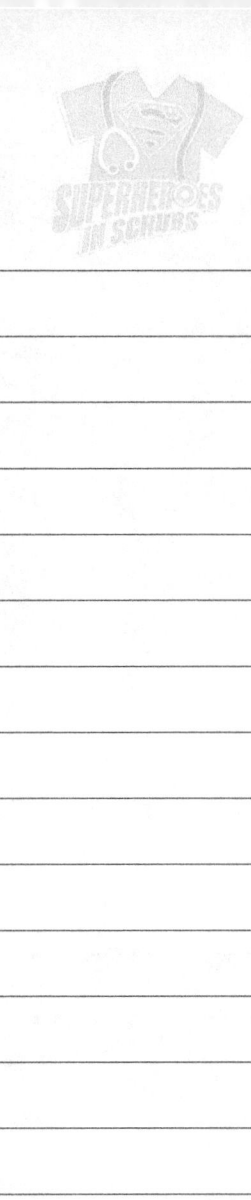

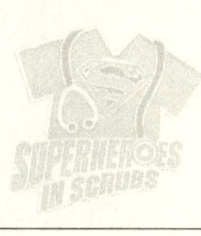

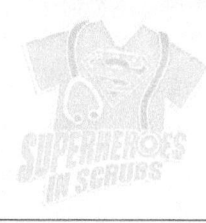

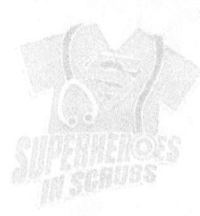

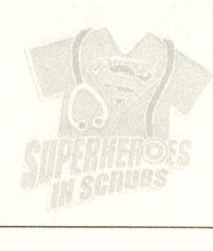

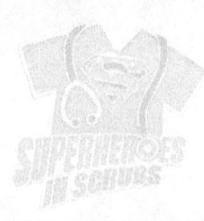

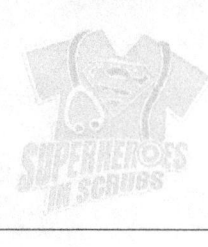

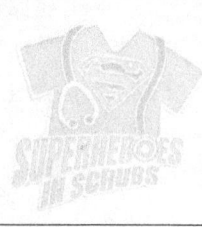

www.ingramcontent.com/pod-product-compliance
Lightning Source LLC
Chambersburg PA
CBHW030625220526
45463CB00004B/1424